High Risk

High Risk

Iron Ivan Edwards

Writers Club Press

San Jose New York Lincoln Shanghai

High Risk

Writers Club Press
an imprint of iUniverse.com, Inc.

For information address:
iUniverse.com, Inc.
620 North 48th Street, Suite 201
Lincoln, NE 68504-3467
www.iuniverse.com

ISBN: 0-595-14248-6

Printed in the United States of America

CONTENTS

FOREWORD

The United State Government has recently issued statements to the effect that millions of Americans are obese or fast becoming obese and are at risk of being in poor health. The government is considering placing ads as to what you should and should not eat. It is certainly very commendable that our people in government would try to turn this condition around by placing these ads, if they will do any good. However, there are two things missing for this to work, as you will read in the pages that follow. The FORMULA tells you how this turnaround can take place for you.

PREFACE

If You're In Shape

Don't Read This. Don't buy it. This book is dynamite—but it is not for you. You are already in shape. Being in shape means that you are within five pounds of your ideal (correct) weight and you do one or more of the following:

- Work out with weights for 1 hour 3 times per week.
- Walk 1 hour per day 3 days per week.
- Participate in an aerobics class 3 times per week.
- Play 3 games of racquetball or squash 3 times per week.
- Bicycle for 1 hour 3 times per week.
- Karate or kick boxing 3 times per week.
- Participate in an organized sport such as soccer, basketball, football or softball 3 times per week.
- Play 2 sets of tennis 3 times per week.
- Run 5 miles per day, 3 days per week.
- Swim for 1 hour 3 times per week.

Congratulations are definitely in order for your personal tenacity, regimentation and dedication to a more healthful life. You should receive a national health and fitness medal. Consider yourself a member of a rather small but elite group of people—approximately 12 percent of the population of the United States. The figure of 30 million people is pathetically too small!

ABOUT THE TITLE

If you are overweight and out of shape, you are among approximately 120 million adults! This book is for you and it is designed to make you motivated. Consequently, you might even be a little bit angry at me for continually saying that you are fat and lazy but what is more important—angry at yourself because it is true. Yes, you are fat and you know it. You eat too much and you know it. You eat the wrong foods; the fatty stuff; the sweets, and you know it. You are buying clothes that are too big for you so you can hide your ever-growing body and you know that will continue to happen and you are thinking "so what, who cares." You are also thinking "how does this guy know what I am thinking?"

At this point, put the book down if you are thoroughly offended. Stay fat! Be content with your overweight and weak condition; be stubborn; stay in your shell.

You have read many of the modern fitness books, listened to and seen all the popular tapes about weight training and aerobics conditioning. You have read all about some of the 21,000 or so diets that are on the market. You have been to your doctor, but you do not listen to him. You have even been to a hypnotist.

Nothing has worked for you, maybe for others, but nothing has worked for you. So, why should you try? Why should you read this much less buy it? This is just another socalled magic cure-all that will not do a thing for you. The fact "*You're Too Lazy, You'll Never Do It*", says it all. What a negative statement!

However, maybe, just maybe, you are curious. Maybe you are not too angry to continue to read to find the one thing that is missing in most of the diet books. The one thing that is missing in all the fitness books and tapes. The FORMULA to success of a healthy, fit and energetic life is in these pages. So maybe these few words of wisdom can be your "on button."

The absolute first thing you must do is pay attention! Yes, pay attention to what this author has to say (Yeah, sure, what does this guy know—formula?) Okay, why should you pay attention to this when all else has failed to do any good for you?

The original title was *You're Too Lazy, You'll Never Do It!* It was chosen because it is true of more than 120 million adults in the United States. Some (or a group) are overweight and they will not lift weights, participate in aerobics, walk, run, bike, swim or any other regular physical activity. This is written in the hope that a small percentage of this group will really listen and turn their lives around—maybe even you! If you "get off it" and start up a sustained day-in, day-out program of two things: mandatory proper eating, and mandatory regular exercise. I will have succeeded in changing your life for the better, which is the reason for this book.

Listen to this - Here's what most of you do now: You eat some kind of breakfast every morning. There is a mid-morning snack. Of course, you absolutely have to eat lunch. Another must is the afternoon snack on your break because you are hungry and do not know whether you can make it until dinner. The big meal of the day is dinner. Never pass up that one! Have I missed a snack or two? Do not forget that "raid on the refrigerator." Then, after you have been a galloping glutton for a span of 14 to 16 hours, you feel stuffed and too tired to go on. So, you go to bed. No exercise at all from up to down. No time? Your energy level has been going down and down and you have not really noticed the change (a little bit every day). Part or most of the reason you are tired is that you are carrying around some extra weight without any muscles to help you do this. Let me give you an example: Let us say you are 5'7" and you should weigh 130 to 150 pounds but instead you weigh 250—an extra 100 pounds! Think about it. Could you or would you carry two fifty pound dumbbells around all day, day in and day out, year in and year out? No way! That's what you are doing right now. Even if you're 20 pounds over you still get tired at the end of the day. You cannot help it. You are tired and weak. Listen up, the amazing thing that happens when you start exercising is you begin a process of reversal. A process of increasing your energy level while burning off excess fat. This is where you and the rest of the big group of 120 million others say: "I don't believe this—that I can exercise and be so excruciatingly tired from exercising and still gain energy and burn fat."

Unless you believe in this reversal and learn The FORMULA, you will never start it. You will go on your merry way as you have in the past. You really have given up everything except existing. Listen to this, what if this guy, what's his name? Iron-Ivan is right.

Without regular exercise, a terrible psychological negative occurs. In the very beginning of the increase of your body weight (10, 20, 30 years ago?) you began to be self-conscious about your fat (the big clothing man-ufacturers love you). As you gained more weight (20 to 30 pounds) you began to be downright embarrassed about it. Now you start to be angrily defensive about it. Then come the biggest "cop outs" ever: "I like the way I am." "My spouse likes me the way I am." "Fat is beautiful." "There is more to love." "It is my metabolism." Bull! Pure bull!

Self-esteem got buried down in there somewhere. It can only be brought up by exercise—but not if you stay complacent and do not believe. I know it works. Try it. Those of you who are stubborn will say "Some jerk comes along and says if I exercise I will lose weight, tone up, get strong, gain energy and feel better about myself. I do not believe it. It's some guy that is out to make a buck. They all are!" Well, maybe so, but if this works for you that in itself will be my real reward.

To continue, when you gained so much weight your ego went to heck. Now you do not care enough about yourself to do something about it. More importantly, you do not think anyone else cares about you. Combining this tragic ego loss, ensuing laziness, depression, galloping gluttonies, and definitely a disbelief in exercising, you get someone who is just sitting there, merely existing and presumably on the way to ill health. Ugh! Oh, oh, getting mad? I hope so! Maybe mad enough to really listen.

Who wants to listen to needling? People do not like to hear they are complacent. In fact, nobody likes to be told what to do or when to do it. If you sincerely feel I have you trapped in a corner, quit now. Read no more.

If you have opened your mind to the possibility of your belief in what I am saying—why not go further?

If a few of you will start exercising and stay on it, I will consider this message a great success. I will have done what so many fitness and diet people have thus far failed to do. Why should I care what you do? I care because you and so many others like you do not have what I have. You do not have what my students and friends have been shown and believe in, they know it works: The FORMULA, the way to a better life of fitness and health. I have been able to show my students up close, one on one, but the only way I can reach you is by the written word.

ABOUT THE AUTHOR

The author, Iron-Ivan Edwards, EWT, is the certified world's record holder for circuit weight lifting in a continuous one-hour period. Two people (Steve Ammons and Norm Wirsching) timed and certified Ivan's accomplishment, as well as six other witnesses. He lifted 111.3 tons (222,600 pounds). A total of one year was dedicated to the groundwork for this event.

Beginning in early 1991, Ivan, at age 63, began to speed press for 20 minutes at a time. In an example of this preparation, Ivan pressed 180 pounds with his legs on 3 different leg machines or stations once per second 10 times and rested for 10 seconds. He continued until his body said it was time to quit. This procedure was used twice per week until the weight achieved totaled 74,200 pounds in 20 minutes. After pressing that total with his legs, Ivan added 3 different upper body exercises using 100 pounds for each press. Alternating upper and lower body presses using the 1 second times 10 and 10 second rest, he began this harder stage of accomplishing the total press of 74,200 in 20 minutes. By September of 1991, Ivan was nearly ready. He managed 1,000 presses with both upper and lower body in 40 minutes for a total of 148,400 pounds. On November 22, 1991, with Steve Ammons and Norm Wirsching doing the counting and after the first 20 minutes, he knew his goal was close at hand. He still felt good and full of energy. No water or any type of stimulant was used during the hour. However, a cold turban-like towel was applied to old Iron-Ivan to avoid the possibility of a fainting episode. The tactic worked. With encouragement from Steve Ammons, Ivan pressed the metal 1,500 times within the hour at an average of over 148 pounds with each repetition.

As of this writing, Iron-Ivan is 72 years of age. He is a retired endurance and circuit weight trainer. Ivan is now a one-on-one consultant regarding the proper use of weights as a required method of better fitness maintenance.

While training others in *Rotary Circuit Weight Lifting*, Iron-Ivan has used the same method for himself and in the process has kept in top physical condition. He has shown others, by example, that any individual of any age can become extremely strong, feel very good, look great and, in general, be healthy all of their lives.

Initially in 1987, instead of lifting 3 times per week, Ivan began to lift 6 days per week, which is twice the number of workouts per week required for health and fitness maintenance. He set a goal to lift 3 million pounds in a full year. After attaining this objective, he increased the weight requirements for the next 4 years to lift 240,000 pounds per week and finally to lift 12 million pounds each year.

In 1990, Ivan picked up the nickname "Iron-Ivan." The name stuck. A year later, Iron-Ivan founded the 6,000-ton Club which now exists of a few elite members.

The 6,000-ton Club records the daily amount of weight lifted for 240 days or longer, if necessary, in a fiscal year. Once a person lifts the 12 million pounds in a year, he or she becomes a certified member of the club.

During an interview with Paul Linnmann of KATU, Channel 2, Portland, Oregon, Ivan stated, on national television, "I am sure that someday someone will beat the record." Later he said, "I will show anyone which weights to use, and I will help any person willing to try to break it."

The 6,000-ton Club will be available in the future through your club to advanced weight lifters, but it will require the certification of your club trainer or club owner.

Iron-Ivan's message to both men and women wishing to begin weight lifting: "Weight lifting is like climbing a set of stairs—take one step at a time at a regular pace. It should be incorporated into your life with the thought that if you quit, you will have to start from scratch beginning at that first step."

*An explanation of **Rotary Circuit Weight Lifting**: The method for the continuance of physical endurance and the maintenance of physical strength.
Rotary: Lifting weights utilizing the three major body groups.
  1. Chest, shoulder and triceps.
  2. Back, lats and biceps.
  3. Legs.
Each major group is exercised twice per week.
Circuit Lifting: Moving from one weight exercise to another apparatus and lifting within 30 seconds; continual weight lifting in a rapid manner. Rotary Circuit and/or the 6,000-ton is Club is for the advanced weight lifter only and is not intended for the beginner.

S.A. Wallace

SOME DIETS WORK, SOME DON'T

Maybe you're the one who said, "I lost 20 pounds on the "Fattyme" diet." I can easily believe that. You no doubt did. Good for you. Did you keep your weight down or did you gain it right back (when you went off your diet)? If you are a busy, active person and you either exercise or have a physically demanding job, or both, chances are you did and will maintain your correct weight. That is absolutely fantastic for your continued good health!

Why don't diets work? Why are there so many Americans that are overweight? Those people who are obese don't exercise!

THE AMERICAN WOMAN

For many years women have followed American Society's line of thinking that says women must be thin, even super thin, to be successful in anything they do or attempt to do. If a woman gains some weight, she begins to think she is "out of it" and "can't win". This doesn't happen to all women who are overweight, but it's almost epidemic. This thin thinking is wrong and unhealthy. I would hope that you will start believing that it is how you feel and how healthy you are instead of how you look. Some of the most beautiful women in the world carry a few extra pounds. The point is this-don't even try to reduce the impossibly thin of a clothes model.

The American Muscleman

Also, for many years, men have followed societys' line of thinking that a man should be muscular, even huge. To be muscular is good and healthy provided a man gets regular aerobic exercises along with weight lifting, and providing a man achieves this naturally. To gain muscle requires an extreme amount of time. Hours upon hours in a weight room. Although most contest size body builders will deny this, most of them have to ingest muscle building "additives". Advise: do it the hard way - naturally - keep you good health.

The complaint department is on the back page.

THE SECRET. THE FORMULA:
THREE VITAL INGREDIENTS

Throughout this reading you will find mention of the "FORMULA". The FORMULA consists of three things: CONTINUAL EXERCISE, SENSIBLE EATING HABITS AND GOOD SELF-ESTEEM. You will read that you CAN'T be fit and trim without all three. You will read that you must have all three continually or "You'll never do it!" In the following pages you will read about many of my friends, some 60 exceptional people, and their accomplishments. *They all use the "FORMULA" all the time.*

GENERAL ACKNOWLEDGMENTS

Throughout this writing you will find acknowledgments of exceptional feats accomplished by people who are dedicated to a better quality of life, health and fitness for themselves. All of these people continue to work out on a regular ongoing basis.

My sincerest regards to these many friends, fitness instructors and students for whom I have great admiration and fond memories. I have trained, joked with, cajoled and tutored these people from the beginning of that better life. Quite a few have done the almost impossible on their own and by their doing so have been a direct source of inspiration to me.

For those few of you who feel you are close to a beginning of fitness through exercise and merely need a *push* by hearing or reading about someone who has done and is doing what you should be doing, there is definitely an acknowledgment, a story, about a real person that will make you feel so guilty, so inadequate, and by that will elevate your ego and perhaps give you the needed incentive to do that something for yourself. Chances are most of you will not do anything. Too bad! It sounds very negative, doesn't it? However, it is true.

I have intentionally omitted the names of literally hundreds of others that I have worked with or trained. I congratulate these people. They still participate in water aerobics, play racquetball, basketball, volleyball, squash, or tennis. They lift weights, run, jog, walk, or swim, as do the weight trainers, aerobic instructors, swimming instructors, lifeguards, and sports coaches. It's true that all these people have been a source of inspiration and motivation to me. Their high, always positive, attitudes are a wonderful thing to behold. You would have to be around these people to know what I mean. Marvelous! I would need to write nine more books to cover their story. They are among the most superb people in the world.

First and last: A special acknowledgment.

For my wife, **Connie**, who is my very important better half—my thanks for bearing up under the stress I have created during this writing. Her cooperation, support and input while I have been "off in outer space", often ignoring her, is lovingly appreciated.

From start to finish:

For my special step-daughter, **Shirley**, for patiently attempting to assist me with this frustrating endeavor.

Yes, You Are At HIGH RISK!

(Your Career and Your Health)

If you work in a business where your work requires you to:

Be at a desk for eight to ten hours per day, five to six days per week, and

You drive or bus to and from your workplace, and

After which you take your work-related stress and return to your home and family, and finally,

It's dinner and to your computer or TV and finally to bed,

your health is or will be at HIGH RISK!

In the above scenario, did you walk, jog, or do anything remotely resembling exercise? Probably not. So, yes, you are at risk of contracting a continually pain filled disease or affliction which very probably will be life shortening by many years - unless - you start exercising on a regular basis, not just once in a while but on a steady schedule even when you don't feel like it! It is imperative that you include exercise in you life just like eating and sleeping!

If you doubt this absolute truth, call or write the United States Surgeon Generals' office in Washington, D.C. They'll tell you!

WARNING: See Your Doctor

The very first important word of caution is: See your doctor! Please get a check up before you exercise at home, walk your neighborhood, or exercise at a club. If you have any physical restrictions, you must find out what they are. If you are between 15 and 30 years of age, most likely, your doctor will say you are okay. However, if you are overweight you will probably be advised to lose some pounds and tone up. So do it! If this is the case, you are okay but fat. The only problems you will encounter will be the normal muscle aches and discomforts that come with *start up*. When you get clearance to begin exercise, you may want to walk every day. If you are between 30 to 45, especially if you have never exercised, your doctor will possibly find some reason for caution, probably because you are noticeably overweight. Most likely your doctor might tell you okay go ahead but start very slowly so as not to over work your heart. You may need a special temporary exercise program that will require a trainer at a club with communication between the trainer and your doctor. A temporary program is the bridge between non-exercise lifestyle and a regular beginner's program. The communication from your doctor to the trainer is important because the trainer receives direction as to what exercises to utilize and the intensity of the exercises.

Repeat—Caution: A temporary program is merely step one of many steps for a beginner in the increase of strength and flexibility that you will experience, but it must be utilized. Do not try to start at a higher strength level that might cause extreme discomfort or pain and possible injury.

If you are over 40 and you find you have limitations that are permanent, your doctor may recommend immediate water exercise or even water aerobics. In this case, you need to go to a club with a pool and a water exercise program with an instructor.

The older you are and the longer it has been since you have exercised is directly related to how easy you have to be to your body in the beginning. If you go to a fitness club on the recommendation of your doctor and there is no trainer at the club, go to another club where a trainer is available.

BEGINNER—NEVER DID

If you are among the thousands of people who have never exercised at any time in your life until now, you are a true beginner. You probably were a youngster who went through your early years without knowing the importance of exercise. As I have already mentioned, your teachers did not include it in your school curriculum. Your parents did not exercise. Why should you? Sounds hopeless; however, you could be one of a small percentage of people who "break the chain." This group will have the most difficult time of all groups in correcting the bad habit of sitting around. At least you know why you don't exercise; you were brought up that way. Maybe you could change your life with a large dose of determination. As mentioned earlier, see your doctor before you start an exercise program. When he checks you over and finds that you are physically sound, he or she probably will not say you are "soft." The truth is that when you start to exercise, your body will scream at you, "What are you doing to me!?" This period of one to two weeks of making muscle and burning fat will be difficult because you hurt. After your body starts to shape up (hardens up) the screaming will stop. You will be on your way to a much more active and healthful life.

Probably you have already been warned: "Don't do this, you'll hurt yourself!"; this is just one excuse one might give and then not start a program. Here is yet one more hurdle. You have been a couch potato, non-walker, non-believer for a few, maybe many years. You have been told that getting into shape and losing your excess weight will take some time. So, again, you don't start. Too much trouble, who cares. Not just one hurdle, too many hurdles.

Out of a big group of 120 million people, your group of "Beginner Never Dids" would be the largest. An estimate of these who have never exercised in their lives would conservatively be 80 million people. Are these people lost? Are you?

Please hear this: The fact that you don't exercise is not your fault, not entirely that is. Remember that when I say your teachers and your parents didn't exercise, I really should include 3 or 4 more generations of teachers and parents. This "None Ex" goes back almost forever.

Let us suppose that now you are mad enough at me, at yourself and at the system to do something. There's something missing. Maybe you need to read about a person who really can't exercise. This is a very important acknowledgment written for you:

Introducing **Suzanne Shultz**. Quite a woman! She used to run; she loves to run. Running was part of her everyday life. She was a "running fool", as her friends have said. Then the unexpected happened to this young woman. She fell off the second level of her unfinished new house. Don't ask me what she was doing up on the second story except helping to build her new home. Anyway, she fell. She broke her back, among other things. She remembers that time very well. Her lifestyle was completely changed. Let me tell you about her attitude now. Sure, she had a hard, hard time accepting the truth that she could not run anymore, but now she has transferred her positive attitude to others wherever and whenever she can. She is also dedicated to daily use of the stairmaster.

Helping others has made all things bearable. Substitution of thought and action. **Suzanne** helps her daughter help her granddaughter, who is 7, to regularly practice gymnastics and to do strength building exercises, including one-arm pushups. Not only is she building strength, but also character, self-confidence and building in an education for exercise for life.

Sometimes **Suzanne** becomes sad for herself, but she pulls out of the feeling-sorry-for-me mode really fast when she thinks of others who can but won't because they are too lazy. She gets as angry as a minister on Sunday with his sinful congregation. Think about it: she cannot, you can!

Acknowledgment—The 6,000 Ton Club

The 6,000-ton Club has been designed for a few advanced weight lifters who agreed to lift weights 6 days a week and at least 240 days in a full year. Normally, a weight lifter lifts either low repetitions with heavy weights called "Bulk up" or high repetitions with moderate weights called endurance training. The 6,000 is designed for endurance weight training with the added advantage of strength increase. Bulk up is the ultimate for tremendous strength increase and size increase. However, high repetition or endurance such as the 6,000 training gives a weight lifter some size increase as well as great strength increase. I have attained a triple strength gain within two years using the 6,000 program. I also have seen this gain in other individuals within 12 to 18 months. This was an amazing thing to experience for myself and extremely rewarding to see it happen to others. Also very satisfying to me is to find that most all of the people who completed the 6,000 are continuing to lift weights regularly and are doing aerobics or other types of cross training.

The acknowledgments:

Larry Cunningham	6,000 tons	1993,1994
Grant Getchell	7,500 tons	1992, 1993
Phil Morrow	6,000 tons	1992, 1993
Dr. Greg Otto	7,500 tons	1992,1993
Judge Edward Poyfair	7,500 tons	1992, 1995
Howard Romey	6,000 tons	1992 1993,
Greg Speyer	6,000 tons	1992, 1993
Phil Storch	8,000* tons	1992, 1993
Larry Wills	6,000 tons	1995

*8,000 tons equals 16 million pounds and is equivalent to approximately 18 jumbo jets.

ACKNOWLEDGMENT—WOMEN'S 2,000 TON CLUB

After designing the 6,000-ton circuit weight lifting exercise program for men, I realized that there were many women who really wanted to try my one-year program. It was determined, by a few women, that a woman should be able to lift 2,000 tons or more in a year's time. I designed a program quite similar to the men's with some variations or substitutes in weights or equipment used. Five women began the 2,000-ton Club and by the third month, I realized that a 3,000-ton program was needed. In order to include one special lady, I made up a 1,500-ton program. All of these required a commitment of working out 6 days a week and 240 to 260 days of the year.

The one woman that I designed the 1,500-ton program was **Hermie Wirsching** who, upon competing her 1,500-ton year, admitted in front of national television that she was 69½ years old. I believe television newsman **Paul Linnmann** was quite surprised at this revelation. The pride of accomplishment showed in **Hermie's** smiling face.

Sue Pearson and **Sandy Schill** completed their 2,000-tons in the regulation one year. The necessary time to prepare to start the program is from 2 to 3 months. This is the amount of time and numbers of workout sessions necessary to increase the number of repetitions and to increase the weight per repetition so as to complete each program. All the women participants "prepped up" in 30 days.

ACKNOWLEDGMENT—THE 3,000 TON CLUB

The two women who exceeded the 2,000-ton Club are **Carolyn St. Helens** and **Nanette Sears**. Both of these ladies admitted that they needed 260 days to finish. Flushing with the pride of accomplishment, the actual lifting or pressing was 3,000 tons—that's six million pounds in a year! A wide-body jet weighs 870,000 pounds. They each lifted the equivalent of 7 airplanes!

Presently, these women continue to lift moderately 2 to 3 times a week and attend 2 to 3 aerobics classes a week.

Comment on the 2,000-ton Club: *Anyone can do it. No Way! The 2,000-ton Club is not for everyone.*

1 20 Million Americans—The Facts

There are certain "facts" about people in the United States of America, those who exercise and those who do not. These "facts" are shocking, and they are approximate.

You have heard there is only 15% of the people in the US that exercise. Where did that fact come from? No one seems to know who said it. Somebody did and that percentage has been used for a few years. As low a figure as that 15% is, I am sure it would be a difficult task to prove or disprove. I will not try.

There are approximately 250 million people in the United States. There are approximately 50 million children under the age of 15 years.[1] Using these two facts, deduct 50 million from 250 million. This leaves 200 million adults. Multiply the 15% who exercise times the 200 million gives 30 million adults who exercise at a rate of probably 2 to 3 times a week. The balance is now 170 million adults. Furthermore, I have used an approximate figure of 50 million adults who really cannot exercise; the infirmed, disabled, paralyzed, or physically or mentally handicapped. For most of these people, any exercise of any kind might be impossible. May God bless these individuals with an improved and healthful life.

After deducting for the kids, the adult "cant's" and those adults who already exercise, the remainder is 120 million adults who can but will not exercise. This is a staggeringly large figure that frankly scares me. Out of 250 million people, 120 million could, if they so desired, but do not exercise. The percentage of 48% is shocking!

There are a few exceptional people who have included a period of an hour or so of exercise per day, every day of their lives. I have used the figure of 5% of the 48% of those adults who can exercise. This is another shocker, only 6 million!

A double gold medal, the President's fitness medal, and any other medal you wish to add for the people in this 6 million group! These are the people you see running, bicycling, walking, jogging and working out at a club every day. Are you thinking, "Good for him, but not for me?"

A gold medal should be given to each person in the 30 million group. These are the people who recognize the value of sustained good health and fitness. They follow through and workout 3 times a week.

1. Our 50 million children under 15 years of age are in a special group all by themselves because of very alarming concerns. See our schools. Fix it!

OPRAH

How can you give a good first impression on a job interview, a first date or have high television ratings when you are extremely overweight? Today, it is increasingly important to look healthy, fit and look successful which is to be slim. Some people have actually said that fat is beautiful and do not agree that you must exercise and be slender.

Recently, one woman, who shall remain nameless and who looked to be overweight, appeared on national television and really "knocked" **Oprah Winfrey** (who is my favorite talkshow lady) for her successful exercise/diet program. **Oprah** really "turned it on" and lost a lot of weight and inches. I have never met **Oprah,** but I understand that she has stayed with this program and looks fantastic. Running over 10 miles per day is no easy task, but she did it. Not only am I certain that her ratings have gone up because of this "happening", but I am also certain she feels much, much better for it. What better spokesperson for "diet with exercise."

As for the woman who disagrees with "thin", I am sure I will receive a scathing letter from her because I am calling her fat. She will have to wait a long time to get a reply from me. Fat is fat and lazy is lazy. How can you defend fat and lazy? You can't!

Good for you, **Oprah.** Keep it going! Don't let the fat lady get to you. She has the problem, not you.

I feel empathy, not sympathy for people who are overweight, which means I understand your situation, but I can't agree that it is right for any person to "scorch" someone who succeeded in changing so dramatically to become as trim as **Oprah** has.

It is time for that overweight person to shut up and start on The FORMULA. But you won't, will you?

NIKE—MY FAVORITE SAYING

Nike, the giant of the sports apparel and equipment industry, has said, "Just Do It!" Simple! Short and to the point! Powerful! To me it says it all. I don't know if someone within the **Nike** Corporation personally told **Oprah** or any one of my friends to "Just Do It", but I am certain that these words have been a strong motivator for them to achieve their goals.

I would say it a thousand times to you if that would get you to "Just Do It!."

Why You Won't Exercise—The Excuses

Over many years in the fitness club business I have heard them all. The literally dozens of reasons why a person cannot exercise. Some excuses were actually believable!

Most excuses are just excuses. You may find that you have stated any one or more of the following to someone who had listened with only one ear while that very same person was thinking up his or her own special reason so as not to be outdone. These reasons are seemingly endless in number and because of that, I have written about a very few. You might find them entertaining.

The absolute number one reason you do not exercise is: "I'm too busy, I don't have time." What a lot of bunk! It is apparent that this excuse really works to keep you out of the fitness club. It is believable! You come up with a hundred things you have to do today in order to lie to yourself that you do not have time. The truth is harder to embrace than this one. It is easier to say, "I barely have time to get to work"; or "By the time I get the kids off to school, it is time to head for work"; or "I had to go grocery shopping, we were out of food"; or "I had to get the car washed"; or "I had company over"; or "When I get off work I pick up the kids and go home to fix dinner"; or "I had to do the wash"; or "I have to work overtime all the time"; or "My work is so demanding." I could go on and on with this one but all of the excuses evolving from "I don't have time" are still just that—excuses!

You have gone on this way (and getting heavier) all of your adult life. Probably, you will continue to lie to yourself the rest of your busy life until you really can't do anything. Could I be wrong? Will you be an exception?

After you have used up all or most all of the "I don't have time" excuses and no one believes you anymore, and you're still gaining pounds and inches, you probably have tried or will try "I haven't been feeling well lately." That's a good one. There can be so many ills, aches and pains that are real (or imagined) that you can use to keep from going to a fitness club or for that matter, merely going outside and walking a mile or so. "I can't seem to shake this cold." "I have been running a bit of a temperature." "I think I have the flu." Nobody knows that you are stretching the truth—except you. The real truth is that you have the tired lazys, but if you are like the big group, you will continue to come up with some lie not to exercise. Or will you?

The next excuse is a dilly, "I am too tired." I cannot relate how many times I have heard this one. Why people continue to use it I will never know. It is not too believable. "When I get up in the morning, I am too tired." "When I get off work"; "When I break for lunch"; "This is Saturday I am too tired—I had better rest"; "This is Sunday, I am too tired, I think I will watch TV."

The funny part of using *I'm tired* as a reason for not exercising is that probably the person saying this is really tired. You may be one who experiences this kind of tired feeling. It is called the "blahs." You are flat. You feel down. Yes, you have the blahs! Only exercise can cure this, but you probably won't listen to me. Or will you?

One of the more commonly used excuses for not going to a fitness club is "I'll have to take off a few pounds first." This one is out in left field somewhere. The person saying this is dreaming. How can you start losing weight without burning calories at a faster rate than you take them in? If you expend more calories than you ingest, without exercise, you would nearly starve yourself. Not good! Use common sense in your eating habits, put on loose clothes and get to a club. Go run, go walk—burn it! But you won't, you're too lazy! Will you be the exception and start?

Get this one; this is funny. Your spouse says "I like you the way you are." Your spouse doesn't mean it and with the most sincere look, gives you the solace that you need. You really don't believe it either, but it sounds good. You're fat and out of condition and you know it, but those sweet words from someone else gives you support for your excuse (to do nothing). So you have been pacified. Ridiculous!

Tag this one to the last: "There's more of me to love." Oh, boy! Not commonly used, this excuse is meant to be a bit of humor and helps you to avoid the inevitable.

The next excuse for not getting in shape is one that is also comical and bordering on the ridiculous, "Going to a fitness club costs too much money." "I can't afford it." "Club dues won't fit into our budget." For some time now, maybe years and years, you have never considered exercise important (you and 120 million others) and have never thought of including fitness in your daily living or in your monthly budget. This excuse is not even a good excuse! I do not particularly want to give this any more print space. I will tell you why. You pay your bills; your home, car, utilities, cable TV, clothing, credit cards, doctor, dentist, insurance, food and household supplies and because you are too lazy you don't pay your club dues. Maybe you have paid for your home and cars, all you have is your utilities and taxes and after your health goes to pot you will say, "I should have! I should have gone!"

This is excuse number funny. Funny because you would think that people would think before moving their mouths. I have actually heard this one many times: "I would have to buy new clothes and clothes cost money. I can't do that!" Boy! What a cop out! For all I know you may have used this one. Years ago when you weighed what you were supposed to weigh, things were fine. When you bought clothes for yourself, you did it because you merely wanted new clothes. As the years went by and you outgrew those jeans, pants, dresses, shirts, blouses, coats or whatever and you merely gave the clothes away with the thought "They're too small, I'll never get into them." Never a glimmer of thought that you could lose some weight with effort and keep your clothes. Then what did you do after you threw the clothes away? You bought some new ones because you had to. If you are one of those who has gained 30 pounds or more, you have already bought your new wardrobe (the baggy kind). So what's this talk about clothes cost money, I can't do that? So much for another excuse based on your laziness.

The next and much used excuse is in two parts. One part is probably a lie, and the other is an imagined one. They blend together so that you cannot tell the difference between them: "My doctor said I can't." This is rarely said in these exact words. That's because if your doctor told you "you can't", you would be incapacitated, an invalid, a quadriplegic. The latter or imagined part of this is: "My doctor said be careful; don't do anything strenuous, get bed rest, don't lift weights for now, don't walk for now, don't run for now." "I can't run, it hurts." "I can't walk, it hurts." "I can't lift any weights, it hurts." Further excuses: "After my accident, I can't." "Since I hurt myself—I can't." The list of "I hurts" and "I cant's" is long. Each reason is a lame excuse for sure.

I have heard the many variations of the I-am-sick-I-can't" excuse so many times that they all sound the same—none of them even worth one token on a subway. The serious part of "My doctor says" is this: If you have a minor injury or ache, be sure you see your doctor to obtain the direction you should take, i.e., if you should not exercise for now; if you should exercise with limits, or if you get the green light.

One of the best cop outs is the "I've tried it, it doesn't work for me." Often used with diet only, exercise only and both diet/exercise, the buzz word on this one is the past tense "tried." Somewhere from the time you started your diet and the time you quit your diet, you found the pounds you lost. They came back. This is caused partly because you went off the regimen. You quit eating properly and more importantly, you didn't exercise along with the diet. Then there was the exercise only program. Somebody said you could eat anything you wanted, if you exercise. Listen up! This is somewhat true but only after you have lost those extra pounds. So you exercised for a while, ate what you wanted, and found that you didn't lose any weight you probably gained a few pounds; then you quit. Lazy! The last part of "I've tried it" is when you went on a diet and went to a club because you really listened to one or more exercise/diet gurus that you must do both: "Eat properly, cut out the fats, sugars and excess starches and exercise 3 or 4 times per week." The gurus are correct. You must do both; eat sensibly and exercise. But now what did you do? You quit exercising for no good reason at all. There is no good reason. So when you quit, it didn't work. All you end up with is: "I have tried it, it doesn't work for me." Admit it, you were lazy then and you're lazy now!

This is a cute one: "I don't want to become muscular" or "I don't want to get more muscles than I have now." Anyone listening to these words who has seen or read the muscle magazines might agree with this except that the people who pose for the fitness magazines have worked and worked and worked for years to obtain contest dimensions (and many congratulations to them). For the average person who does work out regularly and continually, the muscle dimensions obtained will not approach contest size for a man or the muscle look for a woman.

Very high on the lame excuse list is: "I haven't been feeling too good lately." Cute! Don't you think? Anyone who has said to me that they don't feel well, opens the door to the question: Why don't you feel good? Keep in mind that I am relating these facts and excuses to the big group of 120 million who can but won't. I presume you are in this group because you are still reading these fantastic bits of wisdom. So, to you, why don't you feel good? Lack of exercise makes you feel that way. The blahs. Have you ever felt that sleepy, heavy feeling upon rising out of bed late on a Sunday morning; had an enormous ranch breakfast (you're still in your P.J.'s), sat down to the Sunday a.m. news, snacked at 10:30 a.m., turned on a football (or?) game with popcorn and perhaps a beer or two; had lunch at 1:00 p.m., changed channels to golf; snacked at 3:00 p.m.; watched a movie with candy in hand at 4:00 p.m.; had dinner at 6:30 p.m.; snacked at 9:00 p.m. and went to bed so tired that you couldn't see straight, hit the door jamb going into the bedroom, then woke up at midnight and raided the refrigerator. Wonder why you feel so tired? Oh! Boy! Most all of this big group will continue day-in, day-out to be in this blue fog because they are not exercising. Are you in the group or will you be one of the exceptions and change your life! Add exercise! Odds are I doubt it.

Get this one! "Going to a fitness club gives me stress, I can't handle it." This excuse is also a *lamie*. The absolute opposite is true. Fact: exercise reduces mental and physical stress. So that you really understand and comprehend, I will repeat it—exercise reduces mental and physical stress! Furthermore, continued exercise (3-4 times per week) keeps stress at a reduced level. Exercise is mandatory.

Here's another laugh: "I won't use a stairmaster or treadmill again; they don't go anywhere. You work really hard and end up at the same place as when you started." I actually heard this statement once and the person really meant it, I think.

Another goodie: What a great declaration: "I work out all the time!." This keeps people from knowing the real truth. You work out sometimes. Big deal! Are you one of these people who are just a little lazy? You still don't exercise enough to be able to say you have a real exercise program. Once you have achieved your proper weight and strength level, you can work out 3 times per week and maintain that level. Any less, you're not working out. You can look at a person and tell how much, if any, that individual works out. I sure can! Encountering individuals with a hangover (at the waist) can be an interesting adventure. They admit to extra weight but insist they work out constantly and all they really need is to diet. Do not believe it! It's a farce in the making!

ACKNOWLEDGMENTS—TRI-ATHLETES

A tri-athlete is an exceptional person who excels in bicycling, running, swimming, and does all three consecutively in competition.

Although you may never do this, what these athletes do for fun just might inspire you. I hope so!

A triathlon is 26 miles of running, which is the same distance as a marathon. However, in a triathlon the distance 2.4 miles of swimming is added. To top that, a distance of 112 miles of biking is also included

The people who participate in triathlons are premium individuals— and made of iron!

Dr. Tom Kovaric and **Richard Wuitschick** both participate in two or more ½ triathlons in the Northwest every year in the over-40 class. If you would like to ride, swim and run in a tri., either one of them would show you how to get started. Both **Dick** and **Tom** do this because they love it and want to stay in top shape enabling them to pursue their careers properly. These very busy people take the time to do Tri's, even though it would be very easy to say, "I don't have time." So much for that excuse.

Bill and **Janet Fallon** continually train together for triathlons and marathons. Both **Bill** and **Janet** have run major marathons: The New York, Boston and London, to name a few. As of this writing, they will run the 1996 Berlin marathon. **Bill** goes even further. He completed the 1995 Canadian Iron Man in the top 10 of his age group (over 50. In 1996, Bill completed the Australian triathlon.

The most marvelous part to all of this—Bill and Janet do it together!

Acknowledgment (Ladies Pay Attention)

If you like to walk, jog or run, take your inspiration from these four women. First: **Mary Ann Scholten,** who at 50-something, runs 3 to 4 times per week, 5 to 6 miles per day. She participates in the local marathons every year. To keep her muscles in shape, she lifts weights 2 times per week. This achiever is in the 3 percent of all adults who work out 5 to 6 days per week. **Mary Ann** does this for two very good reasons: She keeps in shape for her participation in organized amateur soccer, and says she "Feels so good!"

Next is remarkable **Julie Nelson,** another 40-something runner who does this because she loves to run. She gets to her club early each morning, runs 9 to 10 miles in the dark, the rain and the cold. You would think that she is continuing to prepare for the Olympics; however, her main goal is to run 260 days and 2,600 miles a year and to continue to attend two aerobic classes per week. **Julie** says, "I eat almost everything I want to and a lot of it. The almost part is I stay away from fatty foods (even if they say low fat) and sweets."

Marget Baker is a 6-day-per week runner. She runs 5 to 8 miles a day and has a goal to run over 2,000 miles per year, rain or shine. **Marget** loves running and "hates fat." By reaching her yearly goal, **Marget** insures that she will stay slim and trim. When she is not running, She lifts circuit weights and swims in her fitness club pool (who wants to run in the snow?).

Molly Fletcher wants other women to know that you can be 40-something and look 20. She does! Not an ounce of fat. Molly pays particular attention to health facts such as keeping cholesterol down to the proper level and eating sensibly. She is definitely in control. Could you do this? I doubt it. You haven't yet. Too lazy? Yes, even if you have an asthmatic condition, you can still walk, jog and even run, Molly does!

ACKNOWLEDGMENTS—TWO RUNNERS

Young **Joe Crull**, now 65 plus, still runs an average of 5 miles per day, 4 times per week, which totals 1,000 miles a year. **Joe** does this faithfully because, as he states, "I love it!" "Sure it takes budgeting 1 hour a day of my time, but if I can't budget 1 hour per day for my health, I can't budget anything!"

Not to be outdone, **Don Russo** runs 25 to 30 miles per week in the summer and, get this, he runs 10 miles per week in the winter. Hooded and gloved in sleet and snow, this attorney really wants to stay in shape!

AN AWESOME ACKNOWLEDGMENT AT 95!

If you are over 30-something and you still are not motivated to do something in the area of getting fit and staying fit, you might continue this and read about one of the "five percenters." precentors

At 95, young and with that constant smile of his, **Gordon Sherbeck** will tell you that anyone can do what he has done and still is doing. Perhaps this is true but more likely, he is an exception to the rule. **Gordon** is a runner. No, a super-runner! He has run enough miles every day for the last 20 years to have logged a total of 50,000 miles. When **Gordon** reached 85, he slowed down. Instead of running 15 miles a day, he now walks (almost a jog) for 5 miles a day. When you figure that **Gordon** has run the approximate distance of the United States 14 times, you must assume he is a super runner, and an awesome person. When asked about the amount of running he has accomplished he states, "I should do more!"

If you meet **Gordon** and get to know him, you will find that he is happy with the world, the people in it and definitely with himself.

Will you be like **Gordon Sherbeck** and be in the 5 percent group?

ACKNOWLEDGMENT FUTURE DOCTOR

Too busy to exercise? If anyone would have an excuse not to exercise because she is too busy, it is **Lynn Murphy**. **Lynn** not only works for a living to put herself through college but also carries a full study load on her way to becoming a pediatrician. Even with many hours of work and study, she manages to run 30 miles a week and participates in 2 aerobic classes per week as well. **Lynn** says "There is no excuse for not." After receiving her doctorate in 1998, she will be in practice and will be just as busy.

"I will continue running. I will take the time. I owe it to myself to do so." Is being too busy your excuse?

Dancing for Fitness

Yes, dancing is not only excellent for good exercise, but it is also great fun.

Mary Studer, at 60-something has been a fitness club member for many years. She combines 5 hours per week of ballroom dancing with 6 hours per week at her club doing aerobic exercise. **Mary** said, "My dancing and aerobics keep me in the condition I want to be."

When asked what specific diet she uses to maintain her 30-year old body, **Mary** said, "None, I just eat sensibly." When asked what she means by sensibly, **Mary** states "Low fats, almost no sweets or pops, low salt, high protein, moderate carbohydrates, lots of vegetables, chicken, turkey and ocean fish." Really simple! **Mary** is a marvelous motivator.

Acknowledgment—Three Super Aerobics Instructors

With goals to help others to be more fit, to feel better and to look better, there are three special women whom I wish to applaud. Nationally ranked, **Mary Cassidy, Sheila Gooding** and **Susan Ingram**. Masters at the art of aerobics instruction, they teach both men as well as women.

Set to lively music, their various steps magnetically draw their participants (including new club members) into uniform movement, melding together like one single living being.

One cannot help but be fascinated by the groups of 20 to 30 individuals athletically dancing in unison. If you really want to "Get with it", try an aerobics class 3 times a week. What a workout!

Club

The second best advice anyone can give you, after you have seen your doctor and your doctor has given the green light, is to go to a fitness club, join it and start your new life. This advice includes the admonishments you have heard many times: do not smoke, if you smoke, quit! Eat less food, and definitely eat less fatty and sugar laden foods. Eat more fresh fruit and lots of fresh vegetables.

Part of The FORMULA is to eat sensibly and exercise 3 to 5 times per week for the rest of your life. Get that? It's for the rest of your life!. This will work for you and 120 million others who can but won't work out.

Consider this as a basic truth—a given fact: "You must go to a club because you usually can't go it alone." I say usually because the average person in the big group has tried to exercise alone and cannot or will not do it for long.

Let me tell you what happened to you, being that average person. You tried to exercise at home, you even bought one of the best home-style piece of exercise equipment. You used this wonderfully engineered machinery for 30 minutes every day for a week. Then you used it for 20 minutes 3 times per week for 2 weeks; then you used it once in a while for 5 minutes at a time, for a total time per week of 15 minutes. The walls of the exercise room (or was it the spare bedroom) closed in. The room became smaller. Now the equipment just sits, casting an ominous shadow. It appeared to be saying, "I won sucker!" Now you own what is commonly known as new fitness furniture. Looks good. Impressive. A great conversational piece. A friend drops in, you show this friend your new equipment stating that you haven't really used it yet. So what really happened is that you closed the door on it so you wouldn't have to look at it. "Maybe I'll sell it." Well, you tried to sell it and found out that it's worth one-tenth of the original cost. When people buy home fitness equipment, they usually buy new. If you own this type of furniture, you know what I mean. By the way, the price you paid for it is probably 2 years membership in a fitness club.

Another probability that might have happened: you made a vow to yourself to walk one mile every day from your home to a set point and return; the total time is 20 minutes. Why 20 minutes? Because some expert told you that walking 20 minutes 3 times per week is all you need to be fit. So you walked every day for twelve days and just about died. Your ankles were swollen and your calves still hurt. Almost half the time, you got rained on. You sweat so badly you couldn't stand yourself. After the second week you walked slower and only on Mondays and Fridays. That lasted for 3 more weeks and you didn't lose even 1 pound. You became discouraged and quit. You didn't care. You did this alone. Understandable. So you got discouraged. Too much trouble. Who cares?

Then there's the club: "Oh, yeah, I was a club member. That was years ago; I lasted 3 months." You paid for one year up front and lasted 3 months! Let me guess what happened; they took your money with a smile and a welcome. A trainer put you on a machine and gave you several exercises. You went to the club for 2 or 3 weeks. You did all the beginner-type exercises and you were ready to do some more now that you didn't hurt so much. When you asked the same trainer for some help, he or she didn't know what you were talking about. He/she couldn't remember when you started and didn't remember your name. You were almost invisible to them! Rip off! No wonder you stopped going. They took you to court when you stopped paying—they won! You hate them! *They are all the same.*

You, as a potential member, should know that if you are going to pay monthly dues to a club you that you are entitled to all of their facilities. This includes such personal service as having at least one of the staff knowing your full name! I wish to repeat that a normal person can't do it alone. This includes going to a club that leaves you to fend for yourself. That is the same thing as doing it alone. It is extremely important for you to be with someone who cares about you, especially because you are one of those people who really does not care enough about yourself to even bother to exercise (ouch, that hurts!)

Okay, where do you find this caring person? Among your entourage of acquaintances, could it be your significant other or perhaps a neighbor willing to help you run a mile a day? Very possible. How about a good friend? Unfortunately this scenario fails sometimes because your friend will not always want to exercise either. So you are back to square one. You're alone in this—you and 120 million others.

This is what to do—*my friend*—go to a club! (No. I don't own any clubs.) For those of you who have been a member of a club at one time, go back to your fitness center. Insist on the help you require and the care you deserve, and need. If you can't get that care at your club, go to another that will produce. Go to a club with a trainer on staff who will work with you continually, month in and month out. A trainer who really cares about you.

Now, you are not alone. Now you can start exercising. Now you life starts to change. Now you will start to feel better about yourself. Now you will find that your ego is still there, buried but still existing. Your "lazys" will leave you. You will want to go regularly, and you will look forward to it. You will start caring about yourself. There are thousands of fitness clubs in the United States. There are many clubs within driving distance from your home. There is one that will be just right for you. That one club, one trainer/teacher/friend who cares is all you need. I know, and so do many of my students and friends—they know! Spend the money. Take a dollar a day from your food bills and go! Do it!

There are good and bad clubs. There are far more good well-operated clubs than those that are open to provide an income for some club owner. Let's talk about the good ones. This is the club that has been in business at the present address for a few years. One that has reasonably upto-date equipment. One that has top sanitary facilities including shower, lockers and sauna areas. If they have a swimming pool or Jacuzzi, the club owners must provide regular physical chemical check so as to provide you with safe water. If you can see dirt, it is dirt. Pick another club! Shop around.

A good club owner has to be happy reading this. I have previously mentioned the most common failing of a bad club is that they take your money and proceed to ignore you. This is the big hint to go elsewhere. Here's another reason: For those of you who have never been inside a fitness club much less been a member, let me tell you what to look for, or watch out for. First, you walk in and a person greets you with a smile. This is a genuine ear-to-ear grin. It should make you feel great. This person takes you on a tour of the facility. He/she shows you all of the areas that will benefit you. After approximately one half hour of trying out the bright, shiny equipment, you are escorted to an office where you are shown the cost of joining, the cost per month, even down to the cost per visit. Of course, you have to sign a contract. You are asked to dig deep and come up with a year's dues, or if you want to save money, you can be a lifetime member which happens to be "on a special today only." Watch out! This is not recommended. You do not have to sign a long-term contract of any kind. A joining fee is normal. Monthly dues are normal as is a one-year agreement. Those clubs that want more than one year at a time should be avoided. There is a club for you that will give you continual service without taking your money too far in advance.

A little more about the good club: This one is a full-fitness, full-service club that will automatically make you feel welcome as "one of the family" by a sincere, congenial attitude that exudes confidence and professionalism. This club has been in business for a few years and has a staff that will continually monitor your progress. These staff people want you to succeed. You will be pleasantly surprised at how many members you meet who will become your friends. These individuals have the same problems and goals that you possess. Exercising and socializing becomes fun when you are with a friend. You still think I own a chain of clubs, not so. However, it would be a challenge to try to come up with the necessary monies to open new fitness clubs all over the United States. Such clubs would definitely be needed for new members should there be just a small percentage of the 120 million join and begin to shape up. Nonetheless, dreamer that I am, it is not realistic that very many people of the "Big Group" will do this. Chances are you will not; or will you?

CLUB OWNER

Just a note to the club owner or manager. If you have one or more trainers that have a difficult time helping or communicating with your members and they sit and read or work out on their own program most of the time, get them up and active with the members or get someone else who will. The trainer or staff worker should be on a first name basis right from the beginning to encourage a comfortable atmosphere for new members. It is extremely consequential that your staff know your members, be aware of cliquing or favoritism from your staff. Treat all your members equally. New members should be made to feel as though they are *part of the family.* The bottom line is sincerity (or lack of it).

Your success is dependent upon your people continually working with and caring about your members. Check your membership turn over. Is your active file as full as you know it should be?

Your potential new members who visit you for the first time will sense that you only want the buck if your trainer/staff person shows that you do not care. Your guests come in for a reason—not only to check you out but also because they are in need of help. They are silently screaming for it and a *home away from home.* They are saying, "I can't do it by myself!" If you and your staff can show them by word and by action that you care and can really help them, they will join your club—and they will stay. If the reverse happens, they will go away and you probably will never see them again. I will not have to admonish the person who reads this and goes to your club as a potential joiner; they will see for themselves. Time for a staff check?

ACKNOWLEDGMENT—FIVE CYCLISTS

Although I have not had the pleasure of weight training these friends of mine, I still have a great respect for them. I genuinely admire their tenacity, regimentation and love of the good life that cycling gives them. They are an inspiration to me, and I hope they will be for you.

First is **Paul Parker** who will be 73 years old. He looks and acts like 30. **Paul** bikes about 5,000 miles per year and loves his time on the road. I wonder if he even owns a car?

Dr. Alan Snodgrass, a young man of 30-something, rides 90 miles per week on his street bike and usually 30 miles on his mountain bike a week. **Alan** says, "cycling is in my blood. I can't imagine not biking."

Another young man who "feels 30" is **Boggie Bogden**. Over 70, **Boggie** puts on over 4,000 miles per year on his bike. When he is not biking, he swims or plays racquetball or basketball. When **Boggie** was 61, he qualified and finished the Bud Light National Iron Man at Hilton Head, South Carolina.

Is there hope for you? You bet!

If you like the outdoors and you think you would like to bicycle, take inspiration from these guys: **Merwin "Stormy" Storm** at 74, bicycles three to four times per week. He is a fairweather biker which makes good sense for safety sake. **Stormy** rides seven months out of the year, sees a whole lot of country and does about 5,000 miles each year.

After doing five hours of aerobics per week before work, young **Steve Brown** bikes in his spare time after work. Steve does this five months each year and keeps it up because he loves it. He still bikes over 3,000 miles a year.

ACKNOWLEDGMENT—THE ROAD RATS

If you were to start walking rather than running or jogging, you might be inspired by the following group of "walking fools." We call them the Road Rats. They walk in all kinds of weather, five to six days per week. At 5:30 a.m. (yes, that early!) They are out on the city sidewalks in groups of four to eight at a time in the rain and wind. They walk about 20 miles per week, year in and year out—fast and faithful!

Acknowledge the Road Rats:

> **Jeneen Bonnett (Chief Rat)**
> **Rita Huber**
> **Joyce Lowe**
> **Marlene Vanderveer**
> **Millie McDaniels**
> **Sharry Monroe**
> **Diane Lail**
> **Ann Blaker**

Inspiration comes from different people in different ways. Sometimes by word, sometimes by action—but by Road Rats?

RICHARD AND THE 1,000-POUND MAN

A few years ago, **Richard Simmons** did it again. He inspired a young man who weighed hundreds of pounds to reduce to nearly his proper weight. Yet another success story among many that **Richard** virtually caused to happen. He is amazing!

Simmons is one of the lucky few who can and does convey to people that he genuinely cares. He cares enough that he hurts for others. By his caring about this young man, **Richard Simmons** was able to motivate him to do what would be impossible to do by himself.

I am absolutely certain that **Richard** admonished this man to exercise continually (meaning daily) and stay away from the table if he wanted to maintain his reduced weight level and live. After this accomplishment, **Richard** left the scene to do his *thing* for others. Was he thinking fantastic? This is where the lack of self-esteem comes in. **Richard** cared about this guy, but the man did not care about himself. He wouldn't or couldn't listen to **Richard**.

The young man did two things that would kill him sooner than later. Because **Richard** was not there, the man went back to eating enormous amounts of food. He unceasingly consumed as many edible items as humanly possible—and then some! Food probably was and is his closest friend (next to **Richard**). The next element this individual left out of his search for health was a major component to success—exercise! Combined with his low self-esteem and obsession with food, the pounds quickly returned. In no time he had soared to a disgusting weight of nearly 1,000 pounds! Sometime during this increase, the fellow became one of the *Cant's*.

To save his life, the 1,000-pound man had to be taken to a hospital and immediately. Paramedics and other emergency personnel used a special forklift and a wrecking crew to get the man out of his home. His removal required dismantling a large picture window. What an operation!

I am certain that this *event* has saddened **Richard** immensely. Is he thinking, "I cannot be here all the time?"

Simmons is aerobically in excellent shape and has a strong (as well as a compassionate) heart. The plight of this young human being would probably give a normal person great discomfort.

By reading about this extreme situation, I hope to motivate you, to use The FORMULA. Do not let this happen to you!

THE FORMULA (AGAIN)

If you have really been paying attention, my friend, you will know that you need to do three things in order to change the way you have been living.

You must utilize what I call "The FORMULA" if you want to attain a happy, healthy, fit and very satisfying life.

The FORMULA is actually made up of three different factors. They are requirements. They are mandates. The first and the second go together like your two hands, like a pair of shoes, like daylight and the sun. The first: proper eating habits. The second: regular exercise. You must know by now that you cannot be successful in weight loss, weight maintenance, a high level of fitness and health by doing one or the other. You must do both.

Have you really understood what I am saying? There is a third factor—caring about yourself. This extremely important ingredient is a definite requirement. It is perhaps the most valuable component of the three discussed.

The three factors previously mentioned go together. If you do not start to care about whether you live a healthful life then you probably will not. You must visualize a strong, happy and robust life in order to attain one.

There are approximately 120 million people (just like you) who do not care about themselves sufficiently to use The FORMULA I have brought to your attention. You and millions more have become lazy because of the lack of self-esteem. This is why I have said throughout this writing that *You're Too Lazy, You'll Never Do It*! The odds are too great but if you begin, you will join the elite few people who actually mandate the three factors of this "FORMULA" for themselves. They will follow it for the rest of their lives.

Consider this: Tomorrow is one of the most important things in your life. What are you going to do with it? How are you going to live in your tomorrow. Will you dream up another excuse to "not?"

I Used to Do It

"Fact": Thirty million people who can but won't exercise have worked out at one time during their lives. The result being that every one of them quit for some reason known only to the individual.

Earlier you have read some of the most popular excuses given to not exercise. If you are in this group of "Used to's", then probably you have used one or more of those alibis. Not even one excuse, short of a physical disability of some kind, is good enough. All of the reasons used to keep from working out are based on being lazy and a who-cares viewpoint

Being in the "I used to" group should make getting back to exercise considerably easier than if you had never worked out at all.

You already know that the start up aches are really no more than physical discomforts and they don't last long. So there goes that alibi! You already know the benefits of a steady everyday work out routine. You know how you felt. So very good! You were somehow happier. You thought more clearly. Your decisions of everyday life were easier, more positive.

You were one of those kids who was not required to do physical exercise in school. You did not go out for organized team sports while you were in school. You were too busy studying for college exams to bother with something that you were never trained to do.

It is some kind of a minor miracle that, at one point, all by yourself, you began to exercise. Possibly you started because you had a few pounds to lose. You soon quit.

Now, let's assume you are past college age. You are either working out at your career or you are working at home which is a career all by itself. And now you are too busy to exercise daily. You are busy making a living for today as well as making enough money so that you can retire comfortably.

You're busy raising children, teaching them teamwork, something they may not learn in school. Participating in little league, private music lessons, special schooling ballet lessons and so many other fields, you hope to help your child realize his or her individual talent(s). All of this takes time. These are only some of the reasons you quit exercising. These are the reasons you forgot yourself.

If you are close to retirement age, you probably are fifteen to fifty pounds overweight. You are way out of shape. Your total existence is lacking in energy, health and fitness which is the kind of energy you need to enjoy your retirement. You are now or have been working hard most of your life and now when you retire in the non-energy state you are setting yourself up for a big disappointment. You won't have the endurance or possibly the good health that will be required for worldwide travel and, specifically, to go to all of the places you have dreamed about. It is true that it takes a lot of energy when you retire if you are going to do things. Try playing golf, go bowling, play tennis, go to a picnic or go to the beach. Remember when you got out of bed at 6:00 a.m.? Now you're lucky if you get up at 9:00 am., much less want to at all.

Another unfortunate "fact" is that by not including a regular daily exercise program in your life, you will most likely reduce your life span by many years. The number of years left in your life will vary depending on how much you are overweight and how long you have been overweight and how long you have been idle.

This situation is so sad especially when you can correct this condition. After reading this you know all of it is true; however, only a few of you will go out and do something about it. I hope you will, but unfortunately, you probably won't because you're not motivated! Or will you? You did it once before!

RETIRED

Let us assume you are older. You just retired. You are not sick, not disabled, just extremely tired and a little fat. Your thinking is tired. You do not work out; you are lucky you are not in and out of the hospital. You believe that exercise is for the young—neat excuse! You do not want to hurt yourself, another neat excuse! Too often it seems that fitness is identified with the young. When both men and women reach the age of 30-something, some of them think the world stops turning. They certainly think they are old when they reach forty. The majority definitely know they are old and over the hill or at least starting down that path. It is obvious that both men and women accept the aging process very begrudgingly with an anti-fitness attitude. Too bad! This thinking is really a *cop out*. Yes, another excuse to not exercise. So far, you are lucky. You have a constitution of iron. So you think! Wait a short while. If you do not exercise, you will find out that you are not invincible. You think you have a little pooch now? You know what? Most of you will ignore this silent warning and do nothing. You may go on a diet but you won't exercise—oh well! Who cares?

If you were to talk to any of my students, acquaintances or friends, some of who are way over the forty mark, they will tell you that for them old age is associated with good health, more fun in life, more ambition to do exceptional things, a solid, positive attitude, and the absence of aches, pains and very important, fatigue. One young lady who was 69½ at the time, told me that old age is "mind over matter." If you don't mind, it doesn't matter! She works out (aerobics and weights) 5 days a week. She weight lifts approximately 1,500 tons a year.

Seriously, these people, my friends, ignore old age. They know that one day…puff! They will be gone. However, in the meantime, they intend to feel very good, look very good and act like any other young person of 20-something and probably live a lot longer and have a much better quality of life than those people (you?) in that big group of 120 million. Of course, like so many others, you refuse to believe the truth. The truth is you're lazy which is based on the fact that you do not care about yourself. Where did your self-esteem go? Where did the fun in your life go?

A Special Acknowledgment—Norman Wirsching

A good friend of mine for many years is a retired helicopter pilot. He is a very quiet and unassuming person that doesn't think I should make a big deal out of his accomplishments. Norm is a swimmer who knows the value of staying in shape for his health's sake. He usually swam 3 times per week. Beginning at about the age of 65, Norm decided to set a daily goal of swimming 1 ½ miles per day. He increased gradually to 5 days per week with a goal of 400 miles per year. After achieving this very demanding task and feeling so well, he figured why not continue at that rate. Norm swam an average 400 miles per year for 9 years. Anyway you look at this, you see a tremendous feat accomplished. Think about it. That's 3,600 miles! Putting it into perspective—that equals the distance of the United States! So many other people who have witnessed this are truly inspired to continue their own exercise program.

WHO CARES? YOU CAN!

Little or no progress towards a better life can be achieved by dwelling on the hopelessness or the negatives of your past or present life. Preferably, think about developing the good and the positive things concerning your present and future life.

What does this have to do with you and exercise, health and fitness? Thinking that you are really okay is tied in with starting to exercise. Knowing that you like your imperfect self is tied in with the continuance of your daily exercise and the overall improvement of your future life. Sound corny? Hey! It is true! If you believe that no one else really cares about you, then chances are you probably do not care about yourself. If that is true, who else besides yourself will care about you? Who else cares whether you are fat, whether you have fun, smile or enjoy life? Who else besides you will help you to get started and mentally assist you to begin to exercise and continue to do so throughout your life? No one! Now I am approaching the point behind this line of questioning—the reason you do not or will not exercise. You can start on a diet and try one of the new fads you haven't tried yet (maybe the next one will work). You can start exercising by yourself either at home or around the neighborhood, or go to the fitness center that is only 3 blocks away. Without caring about yourself, however, chances are you will quit. Who cares!

You have probably already experienced the old "start/stop" syndrome"—To heck with this, I quit!" It happens to thousands of people, but the lack of self-esteem quickly leads to laziness and that laziness begins a pattern of *who-cares-lazy-I-don't-care* carousel. This probably started with you long ago.

So now the pattern becomes a real belief that *If no one cares about me, why should I care about my fat self?* This thinking is wrong! You are being unfair to yourself. There are 120 million people who think this way. Part of The FORMULA is to start believing in yourself. Begin now! Basically, you are all alone in your undertaking, but that is in conflict with "You are not alone" because there are virtually millions just like you. So only your decision is alone. You have plenty of company. There is only one person who has no legitimate excuse keeping you from a new life, including exercise, and that is you. So you still say "What is there to believe in, I am fat, no one cares, I am getting big around the middle. I just bought 2 sizes bigger than last year." "So who cares?" "I am getting old and I don't care!"

You have read the word "care" repeated many times in this chapter. I will write it one hundred times more if that is what it takes for you to get it. Part of The FORMULA is caring about yourself. So start caring!

Try this: If you have a difficult time liking something about someone you should be closer to, whether it be family or friend, do something about it. Genuinely try to accept the fact that you can like a person 100 percent even knowing that person has faults. We are all human. You have faults and so do I (ask my wife!). Upon accepting another, show that you truly care about the person and what the individual thinks, wants and needs. You will find that your friend or relative will automatically start showing that he or she likes you for caring. An example of this: have you ever stood directly facing a mirror with a frown on your face and had the vision in front of you smile? It's not possible! The reverse of this is if you smile the person in the mirror has to smile back automatically. Everything you do, motion, action or expression will mirror back to you.

So, you want another person to like you? You must first care about him or her. Caring, genuine caring, is contagious, provided this: you must be sincere. If you fake it, the other person will feel it and you will probably never create a solid relationship. The return of caring from the other person will happen. If that return is also authentic, you will start thinking better things about yourself. One notch up with the ego!

A word of caution: there are those individuals who will never be able to sincerely care about you or anyone else. They are narcissistic, super egotists that no one can truly like. It will never matter to them whether or not you care. After all, they have themselves! Do not waste your time and effort on them. Fortunately, this particular type of person is in the minority. Stay away from the person who cares only about themselves because their inability to care about you will mentally weigh you down. Stay clear!

The next step up for your ego is to quit knocking yourself. So what if you are 10 to 20 pounds overweight, so what if you are starting to get gray hair, so what if your nose is too big. There are lots of things you could say about yourself that are negative. They are not worth saying.

After you have decided to quit knocking yourself around, then show just one other person that you sincerely care. Watch the reaction. Soon whatever you did in the "mirror" will come back to you. Hopefully, it will be with honesty. You will be able to feel the validity of the others actions or words. You will be mentally elevated at that point provided the actions and words are honorable.

If the other person is faking, you will know it and by that fact you will know the other does not really care about you. However, it may be your friend has had a bad day, a temporary condition. Let time pass so that the other person's true feelings can come out. This person might be the one with whom you can pair up for walking or jogging. He or she might just be a workout partner and become a trusted friend, day after day.

As I have mentioned previously, finding the friend, neighbor or relative to be your partner to work out with on a regular basis is hard to do. Your partner has other activities with which to contend and they seldom line up with your schedule. It is hard enough for you to go out and walk or jog without having to synchronize schedules with another person. So there is another way to get started on an exercise program. This one eliminates dependence on anyone but yourself. It depends upon your choice of a personal trainer and the fitness club you join (here I go again talking about joining a club!). The truth is—it works! You will have a partner by going regularly to a club that has a professional trainer that you like and who sincerely likes you. The trainer you select (hopefully before you join the club) must be one who genuinely cares about whether or not you lose a few pounds, lose some inches and generally get into shape. This is the kind of partner who will share your desires, your goals and your feelings. Impossible? After being at a club for a short time, the first change in yourself will not be physical, but mental. You will start to like yourself more each day and you will be boosted up one more notch. You will start to enjoy going to your club. You will look forward to seeing your new friend (your trainer). You will begin to meet new people who will give you mental support because they also have your basic interests, your problems and, most importantly, their physical goals are much like your own.

I sincerely hope that I have shown you the reason or reasons why you are overweight, why diets do not work for very long and why you are not exercising. I trust I have given you a way to start. The facts against that happening are overwhelming, the numbers against you are astounding—120 million to one. You can be an exception to the norm and start exercising and shaping up. The odds are that will not happen.

You have heard and seen many of our very good hard-bodied national fitness leaders espouse the benefits of exercise. They look so good you know you can do it, but you didn't. You were moved emotionally for perhaps 10 minutes (maybe). Then you have seen, perhaps even purchased, some very good tapes produced by some excellent aerobics instructors who look so great that you just had to join the millions of others who also bought the tapes. You did not.

What will it take to convince you that you must exercise—you do not have a choice! Oh, Boy! How can I persuade you that you must when you know that you do have a choice, the choice of doing nothing.

The reason I will probably not convince you to exercise is the base reason itself: *You're Too Lazy, You'll Never Do It!* You don't care about yourself. Where and when did you lose you?

While completing the editing and typing of Ivan Edwards' book, "High Risk," I felt as though he was writing directly to me. So much of the text seemed to pertain to my lifestyle; it seemed as though he must have had some inside knowledge about my own exercise discipline (or should I say, lack thereof). For the past ten years I've lived mostly an inactive life do to my lack of energy. I quickly became motivated and started an exercise program. I now am gaining a lot more energy, I'm exercising three times a week and hope to be hiking again with my husband Lou and family, who have been trying to get me to exercise for years. Thank you Mr. Edwards!

Deb Braafladt,
Deb's Secretarial Services

COMEBACK: HOWARD ROMEY, 6,000 TONS

(1992, 1993, 1995)

In 1989, **Howard** was in an automobile accident that was bad enough to have the medics pronounce him dead. They were wrong. He lived. Tough guy! The doctors were certain **Howard** was destined to be a quadriplegic. They were proven wrong. With his own determination and with the love and inspiration from **Howard's** father, Ed Romey, he began a miraculous comeback. From bed to a wheel chair, from a wheel chair to a walker, from a walker to walking on his own. Then, in 1991, at a fitness club in Vancouver, Washington, **Howard** asked me about the 6,000-ton Club. I told him how severe this program is. I told him that he would need to start on a weight lifting program to gradually increase his mobility and certainly to increase his overall strength of every muscle in his body. Howard increased his strength over a year's time to be able to lift the 240,000 pounds minimum per week that would be necessary to start the 6,000. The build up program also had to develop his muscular endurance to be able to lift 40,000 pounds per day for 50 weeks. To make a long story short, **Howard** completed the 6,000-ton Club in 1992, 1993 and 1995. Hundreds of people have gained inspiration and mental strength from this fantastic "return-from-hell" person. This guy had quite an excuse not to exercise. What's your excuse?

THE "CAN'T'S"

In "The Facts" Chapter, I have mentioned that there are approximately 50 million people who cannot exercise. Certainly there is a large percentage of these people who are invalid and confined to bed, wheelchair or walker through no fault of their own. They were born invalid, were in an accident or stricken by disease. I wish I knew of some miracle or magic that would change the condition of so many people; however, that cannot be.

There are some people in this "Can't" group who because of their own inaction of body (lack of exercise) over a long period of time have become invalid. If you are in this group, this message is for you. You are now confined because you did not exercise. You physically went downhill because you did not use your muscles regularly. You did not walk, jog, run, do aerobics, lift weights, play racquetball or tennis or other form of exercise on a 3 times a week program. You did continue to eat and eat and eat and watch television and slept and slept. You became overweight (most of you) and vegetated to finally arrive at the condition where you could not move without pain or extreme effort. If you think these statements are insulting and are written to hurt you, you are partially right. I have not written this to directly insult you but to insult the system you were raised by and it comes out as a slap in the face to you. If you and your parents and teachers and their parents and teachers had been raised by a school system that had mandatory exercise classes every school day from the first grade through the twelfth you would not be in the condition you are now in. I will explain more in the "Schools - Fix 'Em, Now!" Chapter (next).

What can you do if you are in a wheelchair and what I am saying really hurts? Go to your doctor; ask him if you can participate in some form of physical therapy to improve you strength enough to get out of your wheel- chair and further enroll in an exercise program of your own. Find out if you really cannot exercise or what limitation could be put on your program. Your doctor may say walk, so will you? That is a tough one. I would like to see it happen.

During the course of my adult life, I have encountered many people that are considerably less fortunate than myself. These are people who have become seriously ill through no fault of their own. Accidents on the highways as well as in the home claim the health and mobility of too many of us. There is no way to bring back yesterday before an accident; no way for the person who cannot move from the waist down to be able to go to a gym and work out as a "normal" person; no way for bed-ridden people to get up and walk or jog as they were once capable of doing. Then there is the person who did not have an accident, but through the years of a no-exercise lifestyle and eventual retirement, he or she became an invalid.

Let me tell you about a man I know who shall remain nameless. He can get out of bed, he can dress himself, he can feed himself, but he cannot walk normally. He can just barely walk. Over the last few years since his retirement, he has become almost immobile. His legs will not move most of the time. This affliction is not entirely his fault. It is mainly the fault of a failure of our social structure especially our public school system. This guy is a really fine person who has worked hard all of his adult life. When he was a youngster, no one told him that he must exercise every day for the rest of his life. No one told him "If you don't use it, you will lose it." If someone had told him long ago that if you do exercise regularly all of your life chances are you will be healthy and fit and all the parts will work. No guarantees but the chances are good that this would be the case. I am certain this man would have worked out! Every day!

I am saying this to you, my friend, that this is not a remote example of what can happen if you do not exercise. In fact, there are literally millions of people who are in this cannot exercise group of 50 million that could have prevented their disabilities by including a program of exercise in their lives along with the rest of the sensible program called "Eating properly and sleeping enough." You can say "I don't believe this. That cannot happen to me!" Are you certain you should take the chance? It is your life. How do you want to live it?

A WHEELCHAIR STORY

Every day for years, **Jim Horton** has driven himself to a fitness club in Vancouver, Washington. He gets out of his car and into his wheelchair by himself. Because this particular club has the men's workout room upstairs, he parks his wheelchair at the foot of the stairs and uses his metal arm-type crutches to go up to workout on the strap vibrator. **Jim** knows the value of keeping the parts of his body that work in the best shape possible. His dedication to fitness is an inspiration to many members who also have afflictions. **Jim** had polio which left his legs unable to function properly.

Jim Horton's attitude is a wonderful thing to behold. Every day **Jim** enjoys the fact that he is alive and feeling good, and he shows this to others!

WILLIE THE RACE

(YET ANOTHER "CRAZY" WHEELIE)

To know Willie Smalley is a real treat. This always positive and funny wheelchair-bound guy is a pleasure to be around. Willie lifts weights and regularly exercises his upper body, but it's more his attitude than feats of strength that I wish to talk about. Willie is a high techie with a large international firm. People laughingly tell him to keep his speed under 30 while at work.

Seriously, this guy has a racer wheelchair and has achieved speeds up to 55 MPH downhill in competition. Spooky! I'm told he has done a 360 º full turn on one wheel. That should have been on film.

Willie always has something going. He just bought two 1935 cars so as to make one good one and so he can build a street rod. He said to tell you, "There is no good excuse for not exercising. I'm busy, but never too busy to exercise the part that works."

ACKNOWLEDGMENTS—BUFFED!

These exceptional people do their own thing with dedication. They can!

Patrick Mode, a full-time school teacher, takes the time to lift weights 3 or more times a week.. On the weekends **Pat** teaches group ocean scuba diving in the Pacific Ocean. Pretty good for a guy who recently received his Master's Degree in teaching. So much for, "I don't have time." Is he buffed? His percentage of body fat is "minus something!"

Not to be outdone, here is a couple with a super lifestyle. **Terry Ammons** (Steve's better half) who not only runs 5 times a week, but also participates in 5 aerobics classes per week. **Steve Ammons** plays 6 to 8 hours of racquetball and does 3 aerobics classes a week as well.

On top of all this, **Steve** and **Terry** go mountain hiking on the weekends! This is a true definition of *buffed.*

Yet another devoted person who gets out at 5:00 in the morning (that's every morning!) is **Pam "Loner" Lane**. If you are up that early and look outside, you might catch the blur as she races by, regardless of the weather conditions.

If you are an Olympic type and you think you can keep up with her, good luck! She is a miler who runs for endurance. What is her body fat percentage? Low; incredibly low.

Talk about inspiration to get off your chair!

ACKNOWLEDGMENTS—RACQUETBALL

Have you ever thought that exercise is fun? Well, it is if you are a 3 to 4 times per week racquetball player. There are three ratings of players: A, B, or C. It has been my pleasure to be acquainted with several racquetball buffs, whether the good, better or best type of players of the game. No matter what rating, all of these people get a terrific workout, and it is really fun to watch them "battle it out." You talk about perspiration! The aerobic value of playing racquetball is substantial for healthy living. Besides, it is fun!

I wish to acknowledge the following "A" competitors, some rank nationally:

Bob Caswell	Kirk Gresham
Joe Kasper	Steve Lattanzi
Rick Melching	Marty McCarthy
Bruce Nashif	Jerry Olstad
Steve Ammons	Joe Blair
Jerry Moss	
Larry Welton	Joyce Robertson
Lynn Villemeyer	Ken Wake
Joe Pauletto	Mark Hess

You would never exercise alone if you were a racquetball player. You probably will never have high blood pressure or other heart aliments if you play and perspire as much as these people do. What a fantastic bunch!

Our Public Schools—Fix 'Em Now!

So that I can give you some background why there are so many people like you who do not exercise (whom I shall label lazy, and who will probably never get with it) I will have to go back in time perhaps 50 to 60 years. I have to get way off the exercise subject, possibly confuse you and discuss the base root of "you're fat" problem: our public school system.

The way they are operated, the public's apathy about funding education, the levy system, the legal, economic and structural changes required which should bring you around full circle to realize that there must be drastic changes to include mandatory physical education for our children in our public schools without the constant threat of elimination.

A true statement: If you are not taught daily physical education from childhood on, you will not include it in your daily life as an adult.

Our business leaders and our government people in high places generally agree that our public school systems need a curricular and structural overhaul. I do too! You may even agree with this philosophy.

Remember some years back when you were about five? You began school. There were the usual subjects given to make you absolutely brilliant. The Math, English, History, Languages, Reading, Writing and Music were of superior quality, and perhaps other subjects I may have neglected to mention. Although other nations have literally copied our systems, the United States is second to none. Moreover, guess what? You even learned to read and write!

In the 1940's and 50's and even into the 60's, the public school system was adequate enough for most kids to go into the work force and earn sufficient pay to buy a home, car, take vacations all on one income. An individual could even put money aside for retirement funds. Back then the kids graduated from high school reasonably prepared for college, and they were able to make the choice to go to college without going in debt for 40 years. Now, in the 90's, we have an entirely different situation. If a youngster has aspirations of being in the middle class, which means sufficient income to buy a home, 2 cars, raise a family, take vacations every year and, as in the 50's, put money away, it is an absolute necessity that one or both partners have degrees, preferably a master's in their chosen field. Many young people are deciding not to have children early and a great many more choosing to remain childless in favor of successful business careers. Those who opt to have children, must face the stressful situation of finding a safe and nurturing environment to place their offspring while at work. Tough on kids!

Today, one of the biggest decisions a high school graduate has to make is the need to attend college in order to acquire a medium or higher level income. They ask themselves such questions as: "If I go am I ready to borrow the money needed." "Will I be able to repay the loan which will be as large as a home mortgage?"

Through the years, our educational system has changed in an academic as well as a social sense. Nowadays more and more young people go through 12 years of school without having learned to read or write. The system pushes these kids through like an assembly line. How does this happen? To me, this is appalling! To be fair to the conscientious educators who never let this happen, I am sure there are some school districts that work diligently to graduate only the literate.

Why not give our young future workforce a chance? Add three years of income producing classes to the high school curriculum with junior college qualified teachers. A very few of these would be in the high tech business and the trades such as: nursing, carpentry, plumbing, electricity, architecture, secretarial, legal, welding, computer programming, CAD, finance, banking, computerized machining, house construction, road construction and accounting. There are hundreds more. These classes would provide a young person who has just entered high school with the necessary education to begin a career after high school graduation. This addition to his or her education will eventually reward the students with a good solid income for their entire working career. This addition to the curriculum could be incorporated into our public school system which would better prepare our future generations.

Who has control over our schools? Guess! Truancy is a normal fact of life today. In my time even skipping one class was cause for a severe reprimand. I did it once. I was caught and I was "tongue lashed" not only by my teacher, but also by my parents. I never did it again. Today anything goes. Attire is a personal statement, whether it is good or bad. The young kids today want their independence. Oh, yeah! The blind orange head leading the blind! Most kids often get away with wearing almost anything they desire. Pants and jackets big enough to hold automatic weapons that kill other kids, causing many of our public schools to install metal detectors. How do we correct this? As of this writing there are a few school districts that have changed to a uniform dress code. Hopefully, more districts will do the same now that our president has brought out guidelines for a uniform dress code for our public schools. Wonderful! You cannot hide a handgun easily in a uniform. I hope others in charge of school policy agree. Maybe our nations children will begin to study and learn instead of worrying about how they look, what they can get away with, or who they are going to shoot next. Do I sound concerned about our country's future? You can bet on it! I am! Everything that I have to say about "Laziness" in this writing is based on what is or is not happening in our public schools. When you entered high school you found that the school system offered some or all of the organized major interscholastic sports. Your school had a winning football team, baseball team, basketball team and track team. These sports required a continuous training and exercise program in order to keep athletes in top physical condition. The competition was fierce and still is. Then and now, it is a good thing for the select few boys and girls who desired to play in a sport. You had to workout to make it.

However, the physical education for all other students has basically stayed the same, inadequate or nonexistent. No standard sufficient requisite has ever been set for physical education through to the 12th grade in most public schools in the United States.

The standard, now an irrevocable requirement, must be a formal class with a minimum of one hour of vigorous exercise for each school day taught by qualified fitness teachers. This should be five days a week, month in and month out, year in and year out through to graduation of high school. With no exceptions, it should be for all students, not just for the team player.

Many years ago some people in charge of our public schools decided that if there was not enough money to run our United States public schools that physical education would be the first to go. Somebody decided that formal physical education (P.E.) was not a vital part of our lives. That P.E. was not an important part of our education during the formative years, which would provide a young person the realization through repetition of the necessity of including daily exercise throughout their lives.

Presently, there are a few school districts that require only minutes a week of exercise, one of which is in the Pacific Northwest. This district mandates 100 minutes a week. Think about it—only one and one half hours per week! Atrocious! No wonder your thinking does not include mandatory exercise everyday. No wonder you do not believe exercise is important enough to do it every day! No wonder you don't believe in exercise, period!

When I say, *"You Don't Exercise"* I am really saying that you are complacent but it is not all your fault. You were never taught physical education. Your master teachers, tutors, professors and their educators did not teach it either and their teachers did not believe in exercise because they were not taught it. A continuous chain of apathy.

Adding new academic, high technology, trade classes, drug prevention and family abuse classes and probably others during the last few years, has kept physical education at an "if-wehave-time" level.

Unless there is a change in the thinking of the people in charge of our public schools, the future will be the same for physical education in the system. It will be literally non-existent. Too bad!

You, your children and their children will grow up not realizing the real value of physical exercise. Actually, this situation exists today. If you are an educator, you may not agree with all of the following statements, but please follow along with what I believe are the answers.

The one way to create the time for physical education classes in our public schools is to do just that—create the time. Add one hour per school day; make the vacation time shorter. Four weeks total vacation time per year is quite adequate. Show me a corporation, big or small, that gives 4 weeks' annual vacation for all the staff, new and old. It does not happen except for the single few people who have 20 or 25 years with the company. So, American lazy public, how come we have allowed this to continue for more than 60 years? Three months' summer vacation, spring break, Christmas—it has been going on too long. A change should be made universally throughout the United States. The kids won't like this, but they would have to adjust. The teachers and all other support staff will not like it unless they receive the highest possible guaranteed pay deserving of our producers of the most vital national product, i.e., highly educated young people.

Educators will say this won't work because of the economic base of the entire school system. They are right. Every year most every district has a levy vote. If a levy fails, cutbacks occur. It happens too often with critical and chaotic results; school days are cut back, teachers laid off, students stacked 50-60 per class. Just recently, the children in the Portland, Oregon school district were televised going door to door selling cookies to raise money to keep their schools open. This is sick and appalling!

Then, of course, getting to my biggest pet peeve—one of the classes that gets chopped is physical education, if it exists in the first place. This has to change. This is a federal level problem. Our legislators should look at this: Mandate 7 hours of teaching per day instead of 5 to 5½, mandate

280 teaching days including teacher research days. Mandate the increase of pay necessary. Eliminate levy procedures. And very importantly, mandate physical education in every school for the complete school year, every year.

Hoping for these changes will not make them automatically happen. Frankly, I do not think that the majority of legislators that would be involved in enacting the laws necessary for mandatory schooling, including mandatory physical education, will do anything about the situation. The why is that they are also too complacent. They are among the big group of 120 million that can but don't exercise. Can we obtain a majority vote out of the House and Senate? No way! Lastly, on the school system, if these people do not make the positive changes we as a nation will continue to drop in international education rank to near dead last. A nation comprised of an ignorant and fat populous.

While in England in June of 1996, I learned from my in-laws that the British have just enacted a law requiring every child to participate in daily regular exercise in every school in Britain. Wonderful! Good for them!

How is it that we have not done this yet?

YOUR OBSESSION WITH FOOD

Until now, I considered the topic of dieting to be too involved, too complex and really confusing. Almost all of the dietitians and the would-be weight loss experts seem to have new and different diets that claim "If you do this" or "If you do that", or "Eat this" and guaranteed results will take place within X days."

It has been said that there are over 21,000 registered diets in print for you to try (registered with what agency?). There are over 65 million Americans who start a new diet every year! An astonishing figure! There's a lot of money to be made in the diet business. Billions every year!

This chapter was six months in the writing. The research, the volumes of reading, all the confusion. Now I have it figured out. Now there is no confusion. I was trying to find the answers, the truth as to why so many millions of people are "on a diet" and yet are still over weight. It is shockingly simple. It would be a laugh if it were not so serious. If this American obsession (obesity) were considered a contagious disease it would be called an epidemic. Obesity costs us millions upon millions of dollars because of serious medical problems, including cancer, cardiovascular disease, diabetes, gall bladder disease, high blood pressure, high cholesterol and other sedentary overweight based diseases too numerous to mention. You keep on eating too much and keep eating fatty foods and you will probably become a casualty—sick, ill, one of the "cants." Basically, all diets are the same—not complex, not confusing at all. The majority of diets will work "If you work with your diet." Notice the two operatives: the words "if" and "work." The reason that the majority of our adult population is overweight is that people quit and because they don't exercise. People don't "work" at it. An example of this is one that you probably have experienced: you didn't exercise but you went on your diet. You even reached part of your goal by following a prescribed regimen. You lost a few of those unwanted pounds. You were pleased with yourself—you did it! And then you stopped. You went back to the old ways of eating. You were not "working your diet." Chances are you were on a homemade diet only program without including exercise. You felt you could lose weight without the sweat. You were partially right, but the catch was you ate so little each day you were starving your body of the calories, vitamins and minerals necessary to be healthy. No wonder you went back to eating the goodies. You were slowly killing yourself.

What the dictionary says about food: *Food is the general term for all matter that is taken into the body for nourishment., i.e., any substance taken into and assimilated by a plant or animal to keep it alive and enable it to grow and repair tissue; nourishment; nutrient.* **Wrong!** The real definition of food is that it is too often your pacifier, your only friend, your tension relief. It is your *I have nothing else to do* so…It is your *comfort zone*, your *get-rid-of-your hunger-pains* solution. It's your *who cares I'll eat it anyway*, your *I don't care if I am fat, just one more bit won't hurt. I can't help it!*

It is not for me to tell you what to eat or what not to eat. What you should eat is between you and your doctor and your conscience. Down deep you already know which foods are good for you. If by chance you do not know how much and what to eat, go see a doctor who specializes in nutrition and find out what you should eat. However, I can and will give you some health tips in this chapter. Mostly, these ideas are to help you change your eating habits which is exactly what you need to do. These tips will help you clean up your act: or are you too "hooked" on the good-tasting stuff. Here's one: Eat a small green salad one hour before your dinner. Think hard on this idea and try it. A green salad is very filling and good for you. Be very discriminating regarding your choice of dressing. Try lemon and vinegar, no oil. If you do the salad trick, you will find you will not be ravenously hungry when dinner is on the table and you will not hog out and over eat.

Health Joke:

Your hangover has nothing to do with the morning after...

Everybody wants to talk about food. The new restaurant in town, the new recipe for chocolate whatever, the new diet that just came out (number 21,001) the subject of food always comes up in a conversation. The new so-called low-fat quick frozen food dinners for $1.95. You know which ones I am talking about. These are familiar to you. You have bought them in a grocery store and you want to talk about them to your friends. Why is it that they taste so good. They are so good for you and you are still so fat!

Here are some classic food obsession events that occur yearly: The Thanksgiving dinner, the Christmas and New Year family gatherings. These special times are invariably celebrated with a gigantic mountain of food for all of your close friends and relatives to enjoy and over indulge. The high spirits of these festive times can negate the gains you have made in the previous 2 to 3 months of weight reduction. During the summer you did well, you lost those few pounds, then came Thanksgiving with all the trimmings. Of course, you cannot have Thanksgiving without a juicy, fat turkey. You gained a few pounds back. Christmas arrived along with all those wonderfully tempting delicacies. For two weeks you had all the sweet and fatty foods you wanted. Somebody brought over some fudge. It was laying on the table, so inviting! Just one more. You congratulated the fudge maker. You took yet another piece. The cop out: one more won't hurt, after all it is Christmas! The next day after the big hog out, you wished you hadn't.

The holiday event with the absurd amount of food doesn't just happen once or twice a year. This obsession with food is displayed every time company comes over for dinner or occurs every time you eat out. You gained weight this year and you will next year unless: you exercise! You burn the excess calories stored in your fat body! There's no easy way my friend!

Many dietitians have basically ignored the absolute importance and necessity of exercise together with a sensible diet. Throughout this writing there have been many references to diet and exercise separately and together.

To explain "burn" in easy to understand language it is best to go to the dictionary. Look up thermogenesis. Thermogenesis is: *the introduction or generating of increased body heat which will consume calories (fat stored in overweight or obese people)*. The higher and longer heat is generated, the more efficient the burning of unwanted fat. Here we go again—exercise! Once you attain your ideal weight, you will maintain that weight by thermogenesis which will occur only with regular exercise—all year long. Without exercise, thermogenesis will not happen. Your metabolic rate of burn will be too low. You will gain weight.

A Health Tip for the Majority: When you were younger, you were at a stable weight that was probably correct for that time of your life. You gained slowly over the years, a pound here, a pound there. You used to exercise. You became too busy to hit the treadmill. You increasingly became more tired after each day. You began watching TV more every day because you were too shot to go out and walk. Then you bought your home computer. Think of the hours that you have spent just sitting at that computer. The pounds kept coming. What has this to do with a "health tip?" Turn off your TV set! Turn off your computer! Of course, you won't. That would be too much to expect. It would be too hard to do that. You would probably put your food tray away too!

I mentioned that you should consult a doctor who specializes in nutrition as to what you should or should not eat. True. Ask this question: are processed, preserved foods (canned or frozen) good for you? The answer will probably be a flat no. Why is that? Years ago American food suppliers began processing large volumes of food supplies for our armed services such as the "K-ration." These foods could be consumed months after processing. After the proving of this method of food preparation, the new technology was soon disbursed into our public grocery stores: the can-opener-type can; the tab-open can; frozen fruits, meats and vegetables, to name a few. Now we have volumes of six-minute microwave frozen din-ners in our markets. Convenient and fast, many of the preservatives and other chemicals used in the preservation of these foods are harmful to humans when ingested regularly. Generally, most "already-prepared, you-heat-it-up" foods are high in fat and high in cholesterol. What do you think your doctor will answer? Eat fresh, non-processed food if you can. Some (I hope most) doctors recommend exercise every day. Can you do this? I don't think so. You're too lazy!

If by chance you want to show me up, or to prove to yourself that you are not lazy and begin a program of diet and exercise and 30 days from now you step on the scale to find that you have not lost the 30 pounds you expected to lose (you lose 5), don't give up! It will happen!

Health tip: Remember when you were at your proper weight? Was it 10 years ago? Whatever it was, it was a long time ago. Be kind to yourself. Be patient in the time that you will need to return to your proper weight. No, it won't take 10 years, but it will take some months of continued effort on your part.

THE "FORMULA" REPEATED

Health Joke

What do you call an American who eats 18 pounds of ice cream every year? Normal!

I hope I have shown you the extreme importance of including good self-esteem as a key ingredient of the "FORMULA." In the case of the 1,000 pound man, you must see the necessity of thinking this could be you. Maybe not 1,000 pounds, but overweight nevertheless. Will you have Richard Simmons at your side to help you when you need an "ego shot"? You must elevate your self-esteem to think enough of yourself to take care of yourself and to take action and change your lifestyle. Nike says, "Just Do It!" Now you know.

And Finally...

You have read about the achievements of over 60 people, some of who have overcome great odds in order to have a much better life than most of us. I have written about these people to praise them and more importantly, to show you that it is being done. You can do it too!

I wish I could make positive statements to tell you the things that you want to hear; to make you feel good about who and what you are; that being overweight is okay; to falsely encourage you with miraculous sounding words; to lie to you; but I can't do that. Instead, I have called you complacent. I have said so many negative things about you that you must believe by now that you are hopeless. Nevertheless, all these statements are the absolute truth. I make no apologies to anyone.

Another "Funny": Think about one of your last New Year's resolutions. It was the one that you promised to lose 30 pounds by summer. Your chances of doing this were about as good as your promise. You broke your promise just like the year before and like most New Year's resolutions, it was forgotten soon after it was made. Oh, well, next year. Funny? Not really.

However, just maybe there is a positive reaction that can come from this book. If you will not or cannot think about yourself, think about your children, your grandchildren, your greatgrandchildren. Give them a break. Don't wait for our schools to be fixed. Teach your kids to swim, to run, to play ball. Teach them to participate in aerobics. Teach them to participate in a group sport or to take up an individual sport. Teach them the learning of the habit of doing some kind of daily exercise from the time they begin school so that they will absolutely, automatically and continually include exercise in their daily lives along with eating and sleeping. This will help your children in thinking well about themselves and to maintain a high level of self-esteem. Go for it! Get professional help if you need it, but go for it! Your kids don't know it, but they must rely on you to just do it.

Have a good life. See Ya!

If you wish to communicate with any of the exceptional people that are mentioned in this writing, or if you wish to contact me personally to tell me "you started," or even if you wish to tell me "where to go" please write to:

HIGH RISK
PO Box 914
Washougal, WA 98671